Carb Cyclin
Learning to Li\ ...thy Lifestyle

Nicole Harrington

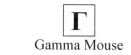

Gamma Mouse

www.gammamouse.com

Introduction

Losing weight can be an extremely difficult process for many people. Even worse is that many people think weight loss is simple, and that if you aren't losing weight you aren't working hard enough. These folks believe that because weight loss is easy for them, it must be equally easy for everybody else.

But dieting is not a one-size-fits-all type of activity. Some of the most serious dieters I've met have been the hardest workers, also, but despite their tremendous work ethic, they struggled to lose the extra pounds.

I empathize with those who work hard, yet don't get the results they are hoping for. I understand the struggle; I understand trying various diets looking for the magic bullet that will finally work for them. This introduction to carb cycling is for these people.

If you are one of those fortunate few who can drop weight easily—first, congratulations—and, second, just following the basic tenets of carb cycling should work wonders for you. For those that have to battle, I hope this guide gives you the knowledge and resources you are looking for.

I have personally witness great results from those who have adopted a carb cycling lifestyle. It is one of the reasons I strongly believe in this diet. I am not saying that the journey will be easy, that this will be like magic, with the unwanted pounds melting away. But I'm confident that you are ready and willing to make the change and to put in the hard work necessary to achieve the results you desire. You have made the first step. Now let's get started on the path to a newer, healthier you.

What Is Carb Cycling?

There is a variety of diets out there that have proven to work. A diet is nothing more than a calorie deficit. Adopting a thoughtful diet or eating less food your body requires will definitely reduce your weight. However, what you eat also hugely determines the type of weight loss you experience. Carb cycling diets are common among fitness athletes for all the right reasons. It not only help you maintain and build your body muscles but also one of the best ways to efficiently burn off fat. For those who are wondering what carb cycling is, I'll take through its sources and importance in an effort to help you benefit from it just like I and many other athletes out there do. Here is an introduction carb cycling.

A carb cycling diet can be better understood as a nutritional approach that involves switching between periods of high and low carbohydrate intake. This type of diets generally focuses on carbohydrate intake because of its key role in metabolic processes related to the burning of fats and building muscles. The main goal of a carb cycling diet is to reduce and refill your muscle glycogen stores, help regulate fat burning and muscles building hormones, increases thyroid activities, and support your psychological state by not needing long periods of low carbs, which can be hard to endure.

When carb cycling, I include the four common types of days that you should also try out: Low carbohydrate/ high fat (LCHF), moderate carbohydrate/ moderate fat (MC-MF), high carbohydrate/low fat (HCLF), and the Full Day Fasts (FDF). Each of the 4 days, protein should be kept high (BW x 1.5 for males; and 0.8 for females). This means that if you are 200lb male, you will eat 300 grams of protein each day; a 125lb female will have to eat 100 grams of protein.

LCHF

This is how I eat on the non-workout days, or the days that I do intervals. On his day, you must avoid eating any starchy carbs and should limit eating fruits to berries and apples. On this day, you should eat healthy fats such as nut butter, coconut oil, olive oil and others, in abundance.

MCMF

You are supposed to eat on work-out days when you lift weights. First meal after my workout, I include between 2-4 palms of starchy carbs. I really love sweet potatoes, and I'm fond of eating them during these days. You should also eat a considerable amount of healthy fats in each meal but not after you've worked out.

HCLF

I would advise you to include this day only if you want to build your muscles. When I replace this day with one of my Moderate Carbohydrates/ Moderate Fat Days once in a week, the result is impressive. It works best and effectively on the day of your hardest workout (full body workout or heavy lower body-lifts).

FDF

Just like the day suggests, Full Day Fasts is self-explanatory. I eat nothing on this day, and i don't visit the gym. I also sip on a greens drink and BCAAs (BW x 0.2 grams) throughout the day. Find some work to do on this day since you are free to be productive.

The Benefits of Carb Cycling

Many people think that losing weight means going without a lot of foods, and the foods that you're not supposed to eat, to many people's minds, are those that provide a lot of carbohydrates. This seems to be a reaction to the "carbo loading" and exercising craze of about 15 years ago. The problem with this thinking is that it's just wrong.

I need to have caloric intake in proteins, fats, and carbohydrates; if I get out of balance with these, I could jeopardize our health. But, there's still the problem of losing weight--and yes, many people truly do need to lose weight. One great solution to this problem is to use carb cycling.

Carb cycling has been successfully used by athletes and physical fitness trainers. It involves discipline with eating, but you don't starve, you eat tasty foods, you get plenty of nutrition, you have lots of energy, and--you lose unwanted weight and keep it off, and lose it faster than you will with the usual "diets".

And, since you'll be getting plenty of carbs with carb cycling, you'll have plenty of mental energy: see, the brain is fueled by glucose, which comes from carbs; and the brain takes its energy before every other part of the body does.

The carb cycling workout extends for a six-day period. It gets repeated over and over every week until you hit your target weight. It will involve first eating carbs that are fibrous--foods like asparagus, squash, zucchini, peppers, and cucumbers--and then, after three days, switching off an loading up on carbs which are rich with starch for three days--foodstuffs like red beans, corn, pasta, potatoes, tomatoes, and yams.

When you're doing carb cycling, you do NOT eat NOTHING BUT carbs. Your daily meals--and there are five or six medium sized ones, not just three large ones--also almost always contain protein, and you also get plenty of water. What matters with carb cycling is the KIND of carbs you eat at certain times.

You see, for the first three days, you are deliberately depleting your body of nearly all of its carbs (you're feeding on them, yes, but the fiber and the water flush out your body rather than being stored, by the end of three day cycle, you have burned off more carbs than you have taken in); then, when you are at the whisk of catabolism, you start off in on a three-day carbo-loading cycle.

By eating five to six times a day, you have to keeps your body's metabolism checked, and it speeded up; this is the beginning of how you lose weight with carb cycling.

Carb cycling requires engagement into an exercise regimen, not the light one. During three day workout when you are eating the fiber carbs only, you are involved in the aerobic exercising: you'll be jogging, distance running, biking, and playing racquetball.

The three days after that, you can still do some of those workouts (if you choose), but you tone them down--you only jog or run two miles instead of six to 10, for instance. You should also incorporate an anaerobic training in two of these starch-carb days. An Anaerobic workouts needs to be carried out for about 12 minutes a day and are greatly strengthened by the lungs and heart, this also enhances the metabolism process

Carb cycling keeps you fit and strong as you're losing weight (1-3 pounds) every week.

Getting Started with Carb Cycling

If you're like most fitness enthusiasts, you've probably been looking for a diet that's both practical and effective. Unfortunately, due to the high degree of misinformation and prevalence of "fad diets", it can be pretty confusing to parse out what works and what doesn't. For now, let's keep it simple and talk about a diet that's been scientifically proven to work: Carb cycling. In its simplest form, carb cycling is a way in which you can strategically plan your carbohydrate intake in order to exploit your body's ability to burn fat.

Conventionally, carb cycling diets feature alternating low carb days and high carb days, depending on when you exercise. On the days that you're more active, you'll eat a diet consisting of healthy, low glycemic index foods such as fruits, vegetables, brown rice, quinoa, and whole wheat products. On your off days, you'll consume little to no carbohydrates, while sticking to foods like fish, nuts, seeds, vegetables, and red meat. Before we discuss why the diet is so effective, let's look at how your body utilizes and stores energy.

When you pack your body with carbohydrates, your insulin levels spike, thus triggering the breakdown of carbs and the intake of glucose (the primary form of energy used by muscles) into cells. If you don't use all of that glucose, your body will store it in the form of glycogen. When your glycogen stores are full, fat storage begins. In a series of metabolic processes, glucose is converted to Acetyl CoA, then linked with other Acetyl CoA molecules to form triglycerides, which are stored as fat.

If your body lacks adequate energy (carbs/glucose/glycogen) at a later time, triglycerides can be broken down to use as energy. How then does carb cycling take advantage of these metabolic processes? Carb cycling is so incredibly effective because you're supplying your body with energy only during the times when that energy will be used as fuel.

You'll be spiking your insulin levels (and thus triggering the intake of glucose into cells) when your body needs it most, which means you'll be alert, strong, and ready to take on your workout.

On your off-days, you'll be resting, so most of the carbs you consume will be stored as glycogen and fat. That's exactly why you'll avoid carbs on these days! By eating mostly vegetables and good fats (omega 3s and 9s such as fish, olive oil, and nuts), your insulin levels will remain low, and thus your fat storage will be minimal. Maybe the most positive aspect of carb cycling is that you aren't "depriving" yourself of anything. The main reason that most fad diets fail has to do with the fact that they're too restrictive.

The dieter is unable to maintain the radical changes demanded by their new diet, and while they may lose a few pounds at first, they'll most likely gain it back in the end. carb cycling allows you to eat the healthy whole-foods you love, while adjusting the timing of their intake. If you're struggling on your low-carb days, you can take comfort in the fact that you can enjoy a rich, carb-rich meal when your body craves it most.

What to Eat and What to Avoid

With new year resolutions, gym memberships are skyrocketing, journal are flying off the shelf for the precious food journals we have been told are so important and of course sneakers and Nikes are practically walking themselves out of stores. All this is all well and good, but without the right information to support your weight loss plans, you are just going to be making the same resolution come next January.

So to make progress and see results, it is time to jump on the carb cycling wagon and head on down to fitness town for that dream body. Carb cycling simply means rotating the amount of carbs you take to correspond with days of heavy or minimal training. I know carbs have been branded with the scarlet letter and the countless no-carb or low-carb diets out there just reiterate the notion that carbs are bad for you but this is totally misleading. It's not carbs that are the problem but rather the kind of carbs you are eating and knowing the right foods to eat and foods to avoid while carb cycling can make all the difference.

Here's why. Carbs are essential nutrients providing the body with energy and eliminating carbs from your diet will more often than not result in a lowered metabolic rate, decreased exercise performance, difficulty concentrating and of course increased cravings and hunger levels.

This is because the body breaks down carbs into glucose and insulin helps body cells absorb it and use it for energy. Insulin tells the body to burn glucose instead of the fat stored in the body cells which is perfect when building muscle and when there are no carbs readily available fat is used as the primary source of energy perfect for losing weight. This is why carb cycling is ideal as it allows you to get the best of both worlds.

There are a few things to remember when carb cycling in order to get the best results. First you need to know the foods to eat and foods to avoid when you are carb cycling so that you don't derail your progress. Complex carbs have the highest levels of glucose and are therefore the best bet. You get these from foods like sweet potatoes, yams, oatmeal, whole grain bread, brown rice, whole wheat pasta and quinoa.

Avoid junk foods as they have higher levels of fructose which is not stored in muscles like glucose instead translating to body fat gains which we do not need. Another thing to remember is to place high carb days on the days you will be doing heavy training as insulin promotes nutrient entry into the muscle cells which promotes tissue repair and muscle growth.

It is also necessary to maintain the amounts of calories necessary for your weight loss. This can be done by decreasing the amount of fats you consume on high carb days to balance the amount of calories from the increased carbs. Protein intake should however remain constant on both low-carb and high-carb days. Keeping a nutrition journal will help you with this so you don't have to keep guessing and is a nifty way of tracking your progress.

Techniques to Get the Most Out of Carb Cycling

Carb cycling is a diet that alternates periods of high carbohydrate consumption with periods of low carb consumption. Essentially, what a person does is cycling his or her carbs in order to achieve a desired result. It works by giving the body the fuel it requires to increase metabolism and create a calorie deficit in order to increase fat loss. Periods are rotated between low/moderate-carb days and high-carb days, with no-carb days in some cases. Below are tips and tricks to get the most out of carb cycling

There is a misconception that consumption of low carbs on a day-to-day basis over long periods of time is good for someone. However, low-carb diets are meant to be temporary diets. This is because they deplete someone's energy and strength, meaning they are not the best approach when trying to shed body fat while retaining muscle. An individual cannot continue with such a diet forever, as the body needs carbs for daily function.

There are also those who believe in high carb diets. As much as these diets help speed body metabolism, they are not ideal for reduction of body fat or weight loss since there is no sufficient deficit to help someone shed the pounds. This is where carb-cycling kicks in. It is an in-between zigzag method that gives individuals the benefits of both a low carb and high carb diet, allowing them to hold on to the muscle they already have and shed body fat. This kind of diet also helps a person to maintain his or her strength, endurance and sanity for as long as the program lasts.

Typically, there are three types of days when someone is carb cycling; high carb, low/moderate carb and no/low carb days. It is worth noting that some days will not go to 'no carb', instead following a low to moderate period and then high rotation. Generally, if someone does three days, those three days are cycled or rotated, although there are numerous ways that a carb cycle can be set up. An individual can also do a low moderate high or low/high.

Generally, the most commonly applied carb cycling approach is whereby someone places higher carb days on his or her heaviest training days, and low carb days low-intensity training days. Such a plan is usually based on consuming food six times a day. Eating five or seven times a day are acceptable alternatives. It is advisable to maintain daily ratios consistent with the chosen meal plan. This means more food per meal if someone does five meals and less food per meal if he or she does seven meals.

The foundation of any carb cycling diet is protein. Assuming that someone is eating six times per day, irrespective of the type of day, he or she will consume a minimum of 1/5, 1/6, or 1/7 of the total minimum required for protein at every meal. The person should maintain dietary fats consistently through his or her plan. Fats will be raised on low carb days and lowered during high carb days.

Thank You!!

I hope you have found this guide to carb cycling to be helpful and informative. I've always thought that knowing where to start is one of the hardest parts of any new diet. Hopefully, you now have a better idea.

I wish you nothing but the best in your carb cycling journey.

A Special Gift for Our Readers!

Thank you so much for your purchase of this book. As a special gift for you we have included one of our bestselling Self-Improvement books: Procrastination: Triple Your Productivity and Accomplish Your Goals written by one of the most well-respected and influential experts on time management, Warren R. Sullivan.

I hope you enjoy!

Procrastination
Triple Your Productivity and Accomplish Your Goals

Warren R. Sullivan

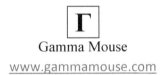

Gamma Mouse
www.gammamouse.com

Introduction

Procrastination. It has a drastic effect on productivity, on our ability to accomplish our goals in life. It can greatly impact our happiness, as we avoid doing something that we are dreading. Yet having to do it still hangs over our head.

Delaying something in order to often do something easier is an easy trap to fall into. Do it enough, and it suddenly becomes a habit. The problem with procrastination is we usually put off more important—but also more difficult—objectives for doing actions that are more trivial. For example, a college student might watch television rather than write a report.

Our time is valuable. It is the one thing that cannot be replaced, unlike money or objects. Yet it is wasted when we procrastinate. Saving this time should be our goal. We need to realize that our time would be better spend on accomplishing our most important objectives. When you have finished those, then reward yourself.

Stopping our procrastination is as easy as changing our attitude and stopping the habit that we have fallen into. In reading this guide, you will learn the tips and tricks necessary to stop procrastinating and start living. You don't have to suffer any longer, you can be happy and more productive, accomplishing all the important goals in your life quickly and easily. But you must take the first step and make a commitment to change yourself. Reading this book is a start, but if you don't act on what you learn change will not come. So consider this a call to action, a chance to truly change your life.

Getting to the root of the problem

Everyone procrastinates. It is part of being human. Whether because of laziness or not having the energy to tackle a difficult task, we choose to relax, to take the easy way out. Understand that not all procrastination should be viewed as bad. Often we need a break from the rigors of our day, a chance to get away from the stress of life. Some goals require great effort and energy to complete, so tackling them when you don't have much energy is realistic.

The line we don't want to cross is when we fool ourselves into believing that laziness is not having the energy to complete our task. Our first step is to recognize when we are being lazy. Clearly, we need to be honest with ourselves, we need to hold ourselves accountable. Secondly, we need to realize that time is our most valuable resource, and that it is finite. No one knows how much time they have, so it is essential to understand how important time is. When you sit down to watch television, recognize that this is time you will never get back.

To borrow a phrase from economics, understand that there is an opportunity cost to ever action you take. When you choose to do something, you lose the opportunity to use that time differently. When you make a choice, there is always a cost, remind yourself of this when you find yourself procrastinating. One of my methods for reminding myself to utilize every minute of my time as effectively as I can is to write the number 1440 on the white board in my office. This is the number of minutes in one day. Whenever I find myself procrastinating, I look at my board, and it helps me refocus on my task at hand.

People procrastinate for different reasons. The first step is to understand the reasoning behind our procrastinating. There may be more than one, but understanding the psychology behind our choices will help us effectively combat them, allowing us to change our faulty reasoning when it arises.

Cognitive distortions are a form of irrational thinking that often lead to procrastination. It is a magically type of thinking. Often we believe that we will be better equipped at some point in the future to handle our task, rather than completely the task at that time.

An example is a person who believes that they need to be in a certain mood in order to complete a task successfully. Or a person may believe that their motivation will increase in the future, and thus will be in a better position to accomplish their goals. Another one that happens in business quite frequently is an employee overestimating the time they have left to complete a task while also underestimating how long it will take them to do it.

If you are putting off a task, because you believe that you will be better suited in the future, realize that you are committing a fallacy. There is no evidence suggesting that your belief is true.

When we are confused about how to complete a task, and the details involved, we may procrastinate giving the reason that we need further instructions before we can continue. This allows us to set the project aside, until we find that we are butting up against a deadline. This reasoning often comes up with perfectionists who do not want to start a task until they are confident in their ability to complete it perfectly. To combat this reasoning, understand that completely the task initially to the best of your abilities and understanding, and then waiting for feedback is much more productive. It is easy to make corrections to your mistakes once the task is completed, as opposed to trying to do the task perfectly the first time. And there is always the possibility that the goal will be accomplished on your first attempt, without the need for further clarification. Don't fool yourself into thinking that if you have additional information, you will be better suited to complete the task. This is a cognitive distortion.

An offshoot of this is avoiding a task because you don't know how it should be done, that you require procedural information. Once again, this reasoning arises most often in the perfectionist, who believes they need to wait for the perfect situation in order to be successful. But look at the great inventors throughout history, who only through trial and error found out how to accomplish something amazing. Imagine if they had waited for the perfect moment, these inventions may never have come into existence. Remember that your goal is to accomplish your task, mistakes that you make can always be corrected. Don't fear failure. Instead, recognize it as an opportunity to learn.

I used to suffer from thinking I needed to take the time, to contemplate and reflect, before beginning a job. What I was doing was procrastinating, convincing myself I needed more information. This was clearly a logical fallacy. Thinking about the job was not going to make me more productive. What was going to make me more productive was doing it. If you believe you need more time to accomplish something, stop and examine whether that is true. Even if it is true, you can start the task now and revise it later as your thoughts begin to coalesce.

We have all had tasks that we had to do that we really didn't want to do. Income taxes come to mind. It is a responsibility, and sometimes that additional pressure makes a task unpleasant. And we are human, we do not want to do things we find unpleasant. We may even fool ourselves into thinking that there will be a point in the future when it will be easier to deal with an unpleasant task. Never make the mistake to think that a task that is unpleasant today will somehow miraculously improve in the future. It is always better to get the unpleasantness over immediately, rather than wait. I am reminded of my public speaking class in college. I always wanted to go first, and I could never understand why people wouldn't want to be first. Most found public speaking uncomfortable and unpleasant, but instead of immediately getting it out of the way and then relaxing, they chose to prolong how long the task would take them. Don't fall victim to this. If you find a task unpleasant, do it immediately; procrastination only makes it worse, and in the process makes you unhappy.

Now the opposite of procrastinating over tasks that we find unpleasant is to procrastinate over accomplishing goals that we don't care about. Finding the effort to complete a task when you are indifferent to the outcome is difficult. Often we may believe that we will feel more inclined to complete a task in the future when we feel more connected with the outcome. Usually indifference does not change, people don't suddenly start to care. These types of tasks often don't get tackled until we run up against a deadline. This can cause us additional stress as we must now take time to complete a task we don't care about instead of tasks that are much more important to us. Understand the cost of procrastinating may not be felt until the future when the task must be completed. Completing the task immediately saves you from future repercussions that you cannot anticipate.

I previously relayed the example of people believing that at some point in the future they will be in a better mood to accomplish a task. They may believe that certain moods make them more productive and believe that they need to wait for when they are in that mood. Recognize that this is an irrational reason you are giving yourself in order to procrastinate. While your emotions can affect your work, this is only generally in the case of extremes. Slight fluctuations in mood will have no effect, so don't convince yourself that you will be in a better mood to complete the task in the future. There is no truth to this.

A more specific example of this idea that a certain mood is essential for higher productivity is the case of individuals who wait until the last moment to start a task. The student who begins to study for mid-terms the night before the text, or the employee who starts an project the day before it is due are two examples of this. Waiting until the last minute to start because you think you are more productive up against a deadline is nothing more than believing that your mood makes you more productive at a point in the future. Don't fall for this procrastination excuse.

An additional reason you don't want to wait until you are up against a deadline is the cognitive distortion in which you overestimate the time you have while underestimating how long it will take you to accomplish a task. If you wait, believing you work better under pressure, you may place yourself in a situation in which you have significantly underestimated the time you will need. This may cause you to rush, resulting in sub-standard work. Or, even worse, you may miss your deadline completely. Avoid backing yourself into this corner where time works against you. Remember that we often believe that we have more time than we actually do.

Another reason people often give for procrastinating is that they had forgotten about a job. Often the reason that it was forgotten is intentional, the task may be unpleasant or one that we are indifferent about. If a deadline is far into the future, it can be easy to forget about our upcoming responsibilities. Or we may believe that we will get to it closer to the deadline. Understand that this is procrastination, and that there is nothing keeping you from completing the job now.

The final cognition distortion I will address is the belief that you don't want to currently complete a job because you are not feeling well, and that you will wait until you feel better. It should be evident how this is very similar to waiting for a specific mood in order to complete a task. Understand that there is no guarantee that you will feel better, in fact, you may end up feeling worse. Granted that people suffer from real health problems that greatly impact their ability to be productive. This is not what I am referring to. Instead, I refer to procrastinators who exaggerate how they feel to shirk their responsibilities. Don't be disingenuous with yourself about how you feel in order to avoid doing something.

Many of these cognition distortions are rooted in perfectionism or in our fear. We are either waiting for the moment to be right, or we are waiting to overcome our fear to do a task we may find unpleasant. Tell yourself that the moment will never be perfect, but it will be good enough to get the job done. Or if you are dealing with fear, realize that confronting your fear and doing the job now, will mean that once you have finished you will no longer have anything to fear. In fact, you will likely feel elated. This is a much better situation to be in than living under a cloud of dread.

Now that we have explored the underlying psychological reasons behind procrastination, our attention will turn to effective methods for dealing with procrastination. By employing the appropriate methods to our life, we will be able to become happier and more productive people.

Recognize the problem

Like with any addiction or problem, the first step is always to recognize and accept that you have a problem. Since you have purchased this book, I will assume that you have identified yourself as a procrastinator, and are now taking the proper steps to remedy this.

Do not feel shamed or embarrassed, identifying and attacking your problems is a noble and brave action. Focus on your self-awareness; stopping procrastination means keeping a keen eye on your behaviors. And making the necessary corrections.

Exercise

I want you to exam your behavior and thought processes. Write down three incidents in which you procrastinated.

Refer to the previous chapter if you want to show why your reasoning was faulty.

Find the root of the problem

Why are you procrastinating? Are you a perfectionist? Is fear keeping you from accomplishing certain tasks? Be honest with yourself. Discovering the root of your procrastination is important. If you recognize the cognition distortions that you are employing, this will give you a hint at the root of your procrastination. While knowing the underlying cause is helpful, identifying your faulty reasoning so you can correct it will have greater long-term gains.

If you are a perfectionist or if fear is holding you back, I want you to take a moment and examine your thinking. Why do you have to be perfect? Does it make you more productive? Does it make you happier? My guess is the answer will be "no". Tell yourself that accomplishing something perfectly is not the goal, the goal is only accomplishing your task. Withhold judgment, jobs are either done or not done. Also, ask yourself is it true that the longer you wait, the closer you will be to perfect? Or would you have done the same job either way? Does the evidence actually support your way of thinking?

The same approach can be taken if you suffer from fear. Ask yourself what you are afraid of? Most people fear a specific outcome. Is it rational to believe that outcome is guaranteed? I may fear dying in a plane crash, so I dread getting on a plane. But what are the chances that this event actually occurs. My chances are much greater of dying in a car accident on the way to the airport, but I don't have the same dread getting into a car. By nature, fear is not rational; it often arises from the fact that we have convinced ourselves of a terrible outcome, even though that outcome may be incredibly remote. Try to look at your fear rationally; assess the likelihood of the outcomes you fear. Then ask yourself: is it really that bad? Surprisingly, our fears are often overstated; they have a tendency to shrink when we look at them rationally.

Exercise

Using the previous chapter, identify any cognitive distortions you have fallen victim to. Can you discern what is behind this? If it is fear or the desire to be perfect, look at potential outcomes. Does it really need to be perfect? Is it a situation that you should be fearful of? Write down the reasons why you believe you need to be perfect, or write down why you should be afraid. Put it away for a day, and then read it again. Do your thoughts appear logical?

Prioritize with lists

Writing down a list is very effective in helping you achieve your goals. But you need to stick with it. Many people write lists, and then don't follow them. Remember the list is to help you stop procrastinating. Once you write the list, don't convince yourself out of following the order you set.

Put the jobs in order of priority, the most important being first and the least important being last. Estimate how long you believe each task will take you. Then multiply that time by a factor of three. Set this revised time as your deadline. The extra time will take into account the possibility that you are underestimating how long each task will take you; it serves as a buffer. The benefit is that if you complete your tasks early, you now have that extra time to do things you want to.

Keep your list close at hand. You can either write it down, or like I do, keep it on a mobile device.

There are numerous to-do list apps that will simplify the process.

Exercise

Write a list in which you prioritize your tasks by level of importance. Decide how long it will take you to do each task, then multiply that number by three. Write down the time needed next to each task on your list.

Divide and conquer

There are some tasks that are so large and unwieldy that estimating how long they will take is an incredibly difficult job. To help facilitate the process, break the large job into smaller segments. These segments should be small enough that you can estimate the time each one of them will take. Make certain you add in a buffer by multiplying each estimated time by three.

If you have a specific deadline, you can now add the time estimations for each of the smaller tasks to arrive at a figure for the entire project. This is a fantastic way to estimate large projects without placing yourself in a stressful situation as the deadline approaches. In fact, this approach is used quite frequently in the software industry for large multi-team projects.

Exercise

If you have a large project on your list, particularly if you are having difficulty estimating how long it will take, break it down into smaller segments. Now evaluate how much time each task will take, keeping the added buffer in mind.

Keep distractions to a minimum

One of the biggest productivity killers in recent years for businesses has been the Internet. It becomes easier for employees to procrastinate when they have other options that are more appealing only a mouse click away. With social media and email, there is always something new happening, and it can be quite difficult not to get immersed in this flow of constant information.

There are productivity plugins that will limit your access to the Internet by allowing you to stay online for short periods of time. If possible, I also recommend shutting down your email program, and only checking it at designated times. One method that is effective is to focus on your task for the first 50 minutes in the hour. In the remaining ten minutes, you can then check your email or Facebook status.

Additionally, a work or home environment can be distracting. People talking, a television playing, and other background noise can make you lose your focus. Listening to music through headphones or using earplugs is effective in blocking out distracting noise.

Exercise

Are you being distracted? Analyze your environment and decide whether you are being distracted. If you find yourself going online to check email or surf the Internet, try to use the 50 minute rule. Browser plugins will also limit your access to the Internet. Research, install, and configure them if you need this level of restriction.

If noise is a problem, buy earplugs or bring your headphones and MP3 player in order to listen to music.

Celebrate your accomplishments

You have completed your task list; time to celebrate. Giving yourself a reward after accomplishing your goals is wonderful way to encourage yourself to leave procrastination behind. The reward can be anything, an hour of television, a movie and dinner out, or an item you want. The point is to make it something you really desire, to properly give you a sense of accomplishment.

Exercise

Schedule a reward for yourself for completing your task list. Make it good. You deserve it.

Take care of yourself

Eating right and sleeping the recommended amount by your physician is essential in helping to reduce stress and anxiety. It is much easier to tackle your task list if you are feeling energized after a good night's sleep followed by a substantial breakfast. Often poor eating habits during the day lead to your blood sugar crashing in the afternoon, leaving you feeling sluggish and tired.

Make a point of eating a balanced diet spread over at least three meals over the course of the day. Maintain a regimented sleeping schedule. Try to go to bed and wake up at approximately the same time every day. Maintaining our sleep rhythms is very important.

Exercise, put it as a high priority on your task list if you have to. This can be as simple as taking a short walk. Exercising has the wonderful effect of increasing your energy, so take advantage.

Exercise

Evaluate your eating and sleeping habits, making the necessary changes. If you are not exercising, start. It can be as simple as a thirty minute walk per day.

Learn to say no

Many of us have the tendency to want to please other people. We take on more tasks and responsibilities than we have time for, causing us to have too many things to accomplish and not enough time to do them in. If you become too overwhelmed, there is a very good chance you will procrastinate rather than tackle your enormous list.

Learning to say no to task of low importance is key. When someone asks you to do something, look at what they are asking objectively. Is this task a high priority to you? What is the opportunity cost to you? Remember that your time is extremely valuable, it cannot be replaced. Time you spend on this task could be spent elsewhere. Unless it is a close family member, the most time I'm willing to spend on a task for someone is ten minutes. If I don't think I can accomplish it in ten minutes (after adding in my buffer), I will apologize and tell the person that I can't do it. Most people understand, they realize that we all lead busy lives. And if they don't, it is only further justification that I made the right decision.

Exercise

Look at your task list. Are there low priority jobs on it that you agreed to do for other people? If so, remove them from your list and let the person know, unless you believe you can accomplish it in a very short timeframe.

Be proactive in obtaining the information you need

During our examination of cognition distortions, we talked about procrastinating because we lack specific information about how to proceed or what our ultimate goal was. The way to avoid this problem is to always ask questions immediately on being given the task. Make certain you understand what your deliverables will be as well as the best way to proceed. There is no harm in asking and getting the answer. It will save you both time and aggravation.

With the advent of cellphones and email, people are generally accessible within a few hours. If the person you need to ask is not available, try to ask someone who has completed a similar task. Asking questions is not only an effective method for curtailing procrastination, it also has a generally positive affect on your life. We live in a society where the majority of people ask too few questions.

Exercise

Examine your task list. Is there a task that you have questions about? If so, contact the person who can answer your questions immediately. Even if it is late, send them an email. Don't wait, act on your questions right now.

Get into the habit

Procrastination is a bad habit, emphasis on habit. Habits need to be broken, and the best way to accomplish this is by replacing them with a new habit. If you have taken the suggested action to this point, you have already started on your way to replacing your habit to procrastinate. But it is only the start. Generally, it is believed that if a person can change their behavior for twenty-one days that change will become permanent.

Exercise

Find a calendar and mark off twenty-one days from today. Your goal is to keep up on doing your task list daily for the twenty-one days. Be aware that you will have to fight to keep procrastination from coming back in. Replacing old habits can be difficult, which means you need to remain vigilant of any back-sliding.

Make tasks relevant to you

Many of the jobs we do are done despite us being indifferent to the task or not enjoying it. The easiest way to combat this is to look at the task and accentuate a positive aspect of it. If you can find a good reason for doing something, it will make accomplishing it much more attractive to you. Think outside the box for reasons if you have to. Maybe completing a task will open up a new opportunity in your life, or allow you to connect with different people. Accomplishing it may give you the opportunity to make new friends.

There are a variety of reasons why a task should be completed. You need to find the one that holds the most appeal to you.

Exercise

Take a moment to examine your list. Are there any jobs you do not enjoy to do? Are there any tasks you feel indifferent about? If so, think of a good reason, one that appeals to you, of what completing the task could mean for you. Try to find a reason that makes you want to tackle the job.

Conclusion

I hope that you have found this journey helpful. If you have participated in the recommended exercises along the way, you should be commended. You have clearly decided you want to change, and that is a huge first step to becoming a more productive person.

Procrastination is not something you need to suffer with, the answers are all right here in this guide. Understand that procrastination can have deep psychological roots, causes that take time and effort to overcome. The best way to accomplish this is to face it head on. If you are a perfectionist, try completing a task even though you may not feel it is perfect, or up to your usual standards. If fear is holding you back, stand up to it by imagining the worst outcome, and then honestly evaluating how likely that outcome will come to be.

Humans suffer from many irrational thoughts, convinced of the truth of an idea even though the evidence suggests the opposite. Recognizing these irrational thoughts is the first step in dispelling them. Once you realize you are being illogical, the thought fails to hold any power over you anymore. Never take anything for granted, continuously question your thoughts, assessing them for validity. This isn't only the key to stopping procrastination, it also leads to a life that is happier and more productive.

I wish you all the success in your journey.

CPSIA information can be obtained
at www.ICGtesting.com
Printed in the USA
BVHW01s1728280118
506540BV00012B/294/P